The Easy Way to
Regain &Maintain

Your Perfect Weight

VALERIE
SAXION

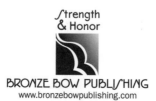

ʃtrength
& Honor

BRONZE BOW PUBLIʃHING
www.bronzebowpublishing.com

BOOKS BY VALERIE SAXION

Conquering the Fatigue, Depression, and Weight Gain Caused
    by Low Thyroid
Every Body Has Parasites
How to Detoxify and Renew Your Body From Within
How to Feel Great All the Time
How to Stop Candida and Other Yeast Conditions
    in Their Tracks

THE EASY WAY TO REGAIN & MAINTAIN YOUR PERFECT WEIGHT

Copyright © 2003 Valerie Saxion

All Scripture quotations, unless otherwise indicated, are taken from the *Holy Bible, New International Version*®. NIV®. Copyright © 1973, 1978, 1984 by International Bible Society. Used by permission of Zondervan Publishing House. All rights reserved.

ISBN 0-9724563-6-8

Published by Bronze Bow Publishing, Inc., 2600 East 26th Street, Minneapolis, MN 55406

You can reach us on the internet
at www.bronzebowpublishing.com

Literary development and cover/interior design by Koechel Peterson & Associates, Minneapolis, Minnesota.

Manufactured in the United States of America.

CONTENTS

ABOUT THE AUTHOR

DR. VALERIE SAXION is one of America's most articulate champions of nutrition and spiritual healing. A twenty-year veteran of health science with a primary focus in Naturopathy, Valerie has a delightful communication style and charming demeanor that will open your heart, clear your mind, and uplift you to discover abundant natural health God's way.

As the co-founder of Valerie Saxion's Silver Creek Labs, a manufacturer and distributor of nutritional supplements and health products, Dr. Saxion has seen firsthand the power of God's remedies as the sick are healed and the lame walk.

Valerie is seen regularly on the weekly Trinity Broadcasting Network program *On Call* that airs worldwide on TBN, Sky Angel, Daystar, and the Health & Healing television networks. She has been interviewed on numerous radio talk shows as well as television appearances. Hosts love to open the line for callers to phone in their health concerns while Dr. Saxion gives on-the-air advice and instruction.

Dr. Saxion has also lectured at scores of health events nationwide and in Canada. After attending one of her lectures, you will leave empowered with the tools to live and love in a healthy body!

To schedule Dr. Saxion for a lecture or interview, please contact Joy at 1-800-493-1146, or fax 817-236-5411, or email at: valeriesaxon@cs.com.

Married to Jim Saxion for twenty-plus years, they are the parents of eight healthy children, ages 1 to 21.

Daniel then said to the guard whom the chief official had appointed over Daniel, Hananiah, Mishael and Azariah, "Please test your servants for ten days: Give us nothing but vegetables to eat and water to drink. Then compare our appearance with that of the young men who eat the royal food, and treat your servants in accordance with what you see." So he agreed to this and tested them for ten days.
At the end of the ten days they looked healthier and better nourished than any of the young men who ate the royal food. So the guard took away their choice food and the wine they were to drink and gave them vegetables instead.

DANIEL 1:11-16

WHY WEIGHT LOSS IS SO IMPORTANT

- **YOU ARE CHOSEN** BY GOD FOR SUCH A TIME AS THIS!
- You have the call of God on your life!
- You have a destiny to fulfill on this earth!
- These are the last days!

You're probably thinking this is a strange introduction for a weight-loss plan. Quite the contrary! Consider the Old Testament lives of Daniel, Hananiah, Mishael, and Azariah, and the profound impact that food had in their lives. The most important reason to lose weight is to empower you to fulfill God's will for your life. I encourage you to read this booklet with an open mind, a tender heart, and an ear to hear our God speak to you about the relationship of your health, your weight, and His plan for your life.

The Bible tells us that the gifts and callings of God are irrevocable or without repentance (Romans 11:29). However, we are the ones who should repent for allowing anything in our lives to hold us back from performing God's will today. God will never take back His plan for your life. He is simply waiting for you to lay aside every weight that so easily hinders and entangles you (Hebrews 12:1). He desires that you "press on toward the goal to win the prize for which God has called [you] heavenward in Christ Jesus" (Philippians 3:13-14). Whatever your calling in life, it is a high calling to be pursued with all your heart.

In Proverbs, Solomon says that the Lord gives wisdom and from His mouth come knowledge and understanding (Proverbs 2:6). We all need wisdom in our daily lives, but many times we do not think of asking for wisdom in small things. There is nothing too small or too big to bring before God the Father. Any prayer asked in faith is pleasing to God. Your prayer may be, "Lord, what do you want me to eat today?" or, "Lord, what is Your will for my life?" The Bible says that He is moved with the feelings of our weaknesses (Hebrews 4:15). And it also says to cast all our cares on Him, because He cares for us (1 Peter 5:7; Philippians 4:6). In other words, if it concerns you, it concerns Him.

So for your first weight-loss assignment, pray and ask the Lord to give you His wisdom. Ask Him to reveal the changes you need to make to achieve your desired goal. If you need some help knowing what to pray, simply pray this: "Heavenly Father, You tell me in Your Word that I am to get wisdom, so, Lord, I am asking for Your wisdom in my life. I ask You to reveal the changes I need to make in order to achieve and maintain my perfect weight. Lord, help me to listen to You and follow Your leading in this area of my life. I want a strong, healthy body, and I am tired of fighting a weight problem. I cast the care of it on You right now. Thank You for hearing my prayer and answering it. In Jesus' mighty name, amen."

THE BIG PROBLEM AND THE GOAL

An estimated 300,000 Americans die prematurely each year of disease caused by being very overweight. Americans eat 300-400 percent more fat than they should, and 800 percent more than they need! Sixty percent of adults in the United States are classified as overweight, depending on the BMI (body mass index, weight/height) cut point used.

A serious health problem exists all around us. We see thousands of people who need to lose weight, yet they are not succeeding and often not trying. The percentage of Americans whose health and longevity are jeopardized by too much weight is escalating daily. It is associated with elevated cholesterol levels, elevated blood pressure, and non-insulin-dependent diabetes mellitus. Excessive weight also increases the risk for coronary heart disease, gallbladder disease, gout, some types of cancer, and has been implicated in the development of osteoarthritis of the weight-bearing joints.

The following guidelines are for general use. Although there is agreement among government and scientific groups about the general range of BMI that constitutes a healthy weight, agreement on an exact range has not been established. The range varies according to age and gender. For example, bone structure and body type play key roles in determining what your ideal weight should be, so factor those in.

Women. Typically, we start with 100 pounds for the first five feet and then add 5 pounds for every inch after that to calculate a female's weight. For example, a five-foot-six-inch woman should weigh approximately 130 pounds. A five-foot-one-inch woman should weigh around 105 pounds.

Men. The guideline begins the same; however, instead of 5 pounds for every inch over five feet, add 7 to 10 pounds. For example, a six-foot-one-inch man should weigh anywhere from 190 pounds to 220 pounds, depending on bone structure and body type. A five-foot-eight-inch man with a small frame may feel quite comfortable at 150 pounds.

I advise people to determine their ideal weight by how they feel. Listen to your body and observe where or at what strength level you have the most energy. Energy is the key ingredient to daily victory in every physical area. Ladies, do you feel more vigor when you wear a size 10 or a size 14? Men, do you feel oomph when you have a 34-inch waistline or when you're at a 38-inch waist? Your body will speak to you. Just listen. It is giving you signals, such as fatigue, poor digestion, high blood pressure, high cholesterol, constipation, joint pain, headaches and the list goes on.

Weight-loss benefits are numerous. Here are a few of the major ones if you drop your body weight by *just 10 percent:*

■ **A healthier heart.** You can lower your cholesterol and reduce your blood pressure through weight loss—two major risk factors for heart disease.

■ **Lower risk of Type 2 Diabetes.** Overweight people are at an increased risk for Type 2 Diabetes, which occurs when your body can't make enough, or properly use, insulin, a hormone that helps convert food to usable energy. Weight loss improves your body's ability to use the insulin it makes, possibly preventing the onset of the disease.

■ **More energy.** Expect to feel better, full of vigor and vitality.

■ **New self-confidence.** Success in weight loss builds your self-confidence and increases your motivation to keep going. When you look and feel better, you're only going to want to improve your overall health as well as continue to shed any extra pounds that need to go.

■ **Live longer and age slower.**

WHAT NEXT?

Now that you have prayed for God to give you wisdom (if you didn't before, do it now) and determined what your weight should be, it's time for goal setting. Remember, you didn't get where you are overnight, and you won't get back to where you want to be overnight either—not safely anyway. Most people have let their bodies go for years, but when they decide to lose weight they want it to happen instantly. It just doesn't work that way. Losing 50 pounds in a month is not healthy, no matter how great it sounds. We need to set realistic goals to accomplish *permanent* weight-loss results.

Let me explain the process of weight loss so that you won't be discouraged along the way to your perfect weight. Initially, you will lose weight quickly as your body burns glucose. Then, as your body begins to lose fat, the weight will come off slower, but that weight loss will be more of a permanent weight loss—not just a few quick pounds of glucose and water.

We want the extra pounds to come off for good, and to do that, we need to do it the right way and get to the root of the problem. No more of this human yo-yo with weight loss again: up some months, and down for others. The human yo-yo routine is never healthy, and it is very defeating to the soul and spirit. So set your goals in accordance with God's plan for your life and for your body type. A good goal to start with is 10-15 pounds the first month and then 10-15 pounds the following months, depending, of course, upon how much you need to lose.

The Muscle Factor

While my purpose is to help you regain your perfect weight, don't underestimate the importance of replacing fat with muscle. While muscle plays several vital roles in the makeup of a healthy body, consider this one. One pound of fat burns a paltry 2 calories a day, while 1 pound of muscle burns a whopping 35 calories. If you gain just 5 pounds of muscle, you will burn 175 calories a day naturally. Over the next year you'll burn 63,875 calories, which equals 18 pounds!

Unfortunately, somewhere between the ages of 20 and 30 we begin to lose muscle if we are not involved in weight-resistant exercise. That loss seems to increase slightly with age, and, correspondingly, our basal metabolic rate slows down (which means we burn fewer calories and usually gain fat). Over 10 years, it is easy to gain 10 pounds of fat while losing 10 pounds of muscle. In that scenario, you still weigh the same, but you have undergone a 20-pound body composition change—probably without even noticing it!

Here's another factor about muscle that you need to keep in mind. Muscle is much denser than fat and takes up less space. If you lose 10 pounds of fat and gain 10 pounds of muscle (no actual weight change), you will probably be 2 sizes smaller! Plus, you increase your metabolic rate by 350 calories a day—the safe natural way.

It's easy to see how the combination of aging and lack of exercise leads to gaining fat. As your metabolism lowers and you don't exercise, simply eating as you always have will put the pounds on. If you want to reverse this inevitable effect of aging, "exercise" must become an active verb in your vocabulary.

FOCUS ON HEALTH AND HEALING

I HAVE HEARD SOME PEOPLE SAY THAT anyone who is eating and exercising right cannot be fat. Wrong! Wrong! Wrong!

After years of counseling others on weight loss, I have come to this conclusion: Most weight-loss problems go far beyond the important roles of diet and exercise. There are almost always root causes that must be addressed first. And if not, the weight may come off, but it will be temporary and health will still be far off.

The greatest root problem I see in people is a state of toxicity—where the body is so toxic and overloaded it cannot metabolize food. So even the right foods are not broken down and digested properly. A low thyroid, Candida, and parasites are also totally disabling to the body's metabolism, but even these can be aided with detoxing.

My point is this: Stop looking to diets and start focusing on health and healing. The weight will follow. Once you are healthy and the energy returns, you will feel like exercising and eating right even more.

God wants us healthy not just skinny and pretty. Remember, He looks from the inside out.

LET'S GET STARTED

ONE OF THE WORST DISAPPOINTMENTS in the world is to set a goal, get all psyched up about it, start on a program, and then crash and burn. We've all done it! Then, that evil spirit of defeat comes knocking at your door with plenty of guilt and condemnation. Here's some really good advice—don't answer! Jesus, the Son of God, is the only person who did not fail His mission. If you fail, it just means you're human. Determine right now that you will keep trying until you succeed.

I'm going to let you in on a secret to help you get started on the right foot—there could be critters living inside your body that are sabotaging your weight-loss efforts! Yes, critters, specifically parasites, and most likely *Candida albicans*. We all have these yeastlike bacteria that coexist in small colonies along with the other bacteria found in our digestive system. It's just to what extent that makes the difference.

The immune system and the "friendly"

bacteria in our intestines (*Bifidobacteria bifidum* and *Lactobacillus acidophilus*) keep *Candida* overgrowth under control most of the time in a healthy body. These bacteria and others make up the normal bacterial population of our gastrointestinal tract and are often referred to as "GI micro flora." They exist in a symbiotic relationship with us and are essential for maintaining healthy intestines and resisting infections. However, when an imbalance occurs in the natural bacterial environment, which can be caused by a variety of factors, then the *Candida albicans* organisms begin to grow at a rapid rate and spread and can infect the body tissues.

These "colonies" of the *Candida albicans* are anaerobic organisms (existing in the absence of oxygen), and when they occur in large numbers, they can release their toxic waste directly into your bloodstream, which can cause a number of symptoms. It is estimated that over 90 percent of the U.S. population has some degree of *Candida* overgrowth in their bodies, and 85 percent of us have parasites.

There are a number of factors that reduce our natural resistance and contribute to

Candidiasis, an overgrowth of *Candida.* These include the extended use of antibiotics (which destroy not only the disease-causing bacteria but also the "friendly" bacteria that help control the *Candida* bacteria), oral contraceptives, low levels of acidophilus and bifidus bacteria in the colon, and unbefitting diets (high in refined sugar and carbohydrates and low in fiber via over-processing). Do any of the above apply to you? Probably, and you don't even recognize that it's wreaking havoc and throwing your body out of balance.

Well, how does this relate to weight loss? It means that if you have this yeastlike fungus in your system, it wants to be fed, it must be fed! You may think you simply have no will-power, but it might just be those critters telling you you need a snack or to snack 24 hours a day. That's what *Candida* does. They crave sugars and yeast products such as candies, breads, and alcohol. These sugary, high-carbohydrate foods and drinks feed the *Candida,* and when you ingest sugar, they thrive and the cravings get stronger and more intense. It becomes a vicious cycle, while all along you naively believe it's you and your lack of willpower!

I encourage you, if you feel there is any chance that you may have a yeast problem, to read chapter 5 of my book, *How to Feel Great All the Time*, or my booklet *How to Stop Candida and Other Yeast Conditions in Their Tracks*. Both contain a Self-Analysis Test to help you discover to what degree you may be affected. Decide if you should start your weight-loss program with a *Candida* cleanse, which will assist you in losing weight, because the sugar and high carbohydrate cravings will disappear before you get started. This will be a big advantage and may have been the cause of your defeat in the past. I offer a new product in tablet form called *Candida Cleanse* that can eliminate the overgrowth as well as help to normalize bowel functions.

JUMP-START YOUR WEIGHT-LOSS PROGRAM

After completing the *Candida* cleanse, you should have rid your body of most of those little critters that make you crave the very foods you shouldn't eat. I say most, because *Candida* will hide in the body, and if you go back to a diet heavy in sugars, starches, and breads, it will start its growth pattern all over again and sabotage your weight-loss success.

Now it's time to move forward with a cutting-edge program that will rapidly rid your body of toxins—fasting. Don't be afraid. I'm going to guide you through a painless form of this ancient miracle that no one seems to understand anymore. In addition to the immense value of detoxifying the body, fasting will also shrink your stomach, which jump-starts your weight-loss program naturally. If this still sounds scary to you, be assured that the fasting program I have designed provides palate-pleasing nutrition that satisfies your senses without eating solid foods.

Fasting means to not eat, but it doesn't mean you should restrict yourself to water only. In fact, juice fasting has proven to be the most effective way to restore your health back to the way God intended.

During a prolonged fast (after the first three days), your body will live on its own substance. When it is deprived of needed nutrition, particularly of proteins and fats, it will burn and digest its own tissues by the process of *autolysis*, or self-digestion. But your body will not do this indiscriminately! Through the divine wisdom of our Great Creator, your body will first decompose and burn those cells and tissues that are diseased, damaged, aged, or dead. In the fasting process, your body feeds itself on the most impure and inferior materials, such as dead cells and morbid accumulations—tumors, abscesses, fat deposits, etc. However, the essential body tissues and vital organs are not damaged in a fast.

In general, three- to ten-day fasts are recommended for health and longevity. The body needs three to five days of fasting to actually begin the autolysis and healing process. A five-day fast essentially clears debris before disease gets started. A ten-day fast works to attack disease that has already begun and often eliminates problems from the body before the symptoms arise. During the fast, the functions of the eliminative organs—liver, kidneys, lungs, and the skin—are greatly increased, and accumulated toxins and waste are quickly expelled. Throughout the fast, toxins in the urine can be ten times higher than normal.

If you have never fasted before, it is best to start with several one-day fasts before moving on to a three-day fast. Do these once a week until you feel comfortable moving on. Then initiate a three-day fast once a month. As a preparation for your fast, reduce the amount of food you consume now and eat only whole raw organic foods two to three days before you begin your fast. I recommend beginning the fast on a Friday evening and extending it through Monday evening. Most people are at home on weekends and can easily do their juicing and cleansing with few interruptions. For many people the second day feels the worst, so it's best to have that on a day of rest. Think of it as a time to give your body a rest, to let it retune itself, and to aid in its healing and weight-loss process.

Fluid Nutrition

Start each day of your fast with a glass of room temperature steam-distilled water. Every day you should be drinking half of your body weight in ounces of water. For example, if you weigh 150 pounds, drink 75 ounces (2 liters) of distilled water each day. Health science consensus currently believes that steam-distilled water is the best for fasting as well as daily use. Steam-distilled water is the only water that actually goes in and pulls out toxins from the organs. It literally pulls out the sludge that gets caught in the follicles of the colon and breeds disease. An added benefit is that you will find steam-distilled water helps curb your appetite.

Juice. The best juices are the ones you juice yourself. Fresh organic veggies can be found at your local health food store as well as grocery stores. Stock up on the freshest you can find. During a fast, my favorite juice is a carrot, beet, and ginger combination. Feel free to use a variety of veggies and fruits. Fresh lemon, cabbage, beet, carrot, grape (including the seeds), apple (skin and seeds), green combos made from leafy greens such as spinach, kale, turnips, etc.—these are all excellent detoxifiers.

Raw cabbage juice is known to aid in the recovery from ulcers, cancer, and all colon problems. However, it must be fresh, not stored. Cabbage loses its Vitamin U content after sitting for only a short time.

One excellent juice blend is three carrots, two stalks of celery, one turnip, two beets, a half head of cabbage, a quarter bunch of parsley, and a clove of garlic. This could be one of the best juices on our planet for the restoration of the body from many ailments.

Another favorite juice preparation is Stanley Borroughs's "Master Cleanser." In a gallon of steam-distilled water, mix the juice of five fresh lemons and a half-cup of grade B maple syrup. Add one or more tablespoons of hot cayenne pepper (at least 90,000 heat units) to your taste tolerance. This is especially good for alkalinizing the body and raising body temperature to help resolve infection and flu-type illnesses.

Pure vegetable broths with no seasonings added are also good. To prepare these, gently boil vegetables, including lots of onions and garlic, for 30 minutes. Do not eat the stew, but strain the broth and drink the juice two or three times a day.

The juices, broths, and water will keep you adequately full as well as provide you with more nutrients than many people get from their normal diets. If you must eat something, have a slice of watermelon. Organic grapes with seeds are also good, especially Concord grapes, which have a powerful antioxidant effect. Alternatively, fresh applesauce made with the skins on and the seeds intact, processed in a blender or food processor, is satisfying and won't significantly disrupt your fast.

A green drink can also be incorporated to your fast. My favorite is called *Creation's Bounty* (formerly *Green Bounty*), which is a whole raw organic food with all the nutrients your body needs. Just add a scoop to a glass of apple juice and you have a complete fluid meal.

A Suggested Daily Protocol for Fasting

- Start with 4-8 ounces of *Clustered Water*™. This will help detoxify and clean out your lymphatic system while increasing the absorption of the nutrients you do take in up to 600 percent.
- Fifteen minutes later take 1-2 ounces of *Body Oxygen*™.
- Thirty to forty minutes later have a *Creation's Bounty* or green drink.
- Prepare your favorite fresh juice combination, which you can alternate with Stanley Burroughs's lemonade drink. If

you don't have a juicer, use the best organic juices from your grocery store.

- Prepare fresh vegetables broth to sip in between juices and/or green smoothies.
- Remember to drink as much steam-distilled water as possible.
- A good liquid mineral supplement will aid in rapid healing.
- If you must eat, remember—grapes, watermelon, or fresh applesauce.
- Rest if you feel weak during a fast. Deep-breathing exercises and frequent showers are pleasant.

WHAT NOT TO DO WHEN FASTING

- Don't fast on water alone!
- Don't chew gum or mints. This starts the digestive juices flowing and is harmful to the system. When your stomach releases hydrochloric acid in the gut, but nothing ever gets down there, is it a surprise that you have a stomachache?
- Don't drink orange or tomato juice on a fast. They are too acidic.

Breaking Your Fast

Fasting brings the body back to doing what it is designed to do, which is for you to accomplish the will of God without the hindrances of fatigue, obesity, and illness. Most people, following initial withdrawal from chemical dependencies (including caffeine and sugar), dramatically see and feel a difference in their health status by day three of a good fast. People commonly feel lighter and more energized and notice improvements in complexion and eye color. These changes indicate you are on your way back to optimal health.

Always break the fast gently. Whole raw organic foods may be used. Nothing heavy or chemical laden should be eaten, such as processed foods. For a powerful aid in rebuilding the immune system before and after the fast, drink Pau d'arco and Echinacea tea mixed with one-third unsweetened cranberry juice four times a day. Lightly steamed vegetables in their broth with whole grain brown rice can be added slowly and used as part of a maintenance diet.

TIME TO TRAIN!

OKAY, WE'RE OFF TO A GOOD START! Now that you have cleansed your body, you can start the remodeling process. It's time to train or *exercise*! There is no way around it, and you probably feel like it now that you're cleaned out and thinking right. There is no magic pill that will keep the weight off or tone your body. You just gotta do it!

When you were fasting, your body was burning stored glucose, and you probably went to the bathroom a lot. Unburned glucose is stored in the body along with water. When you fast, the glucose is used by the mitochondria (think of them as tiny power plants) in the cells, causing you to lose weight as well as to urinate often. This is often referred to as the loss of "water weight," which usually happens rather quickly and is very encouraging. It will be the fastest weight you lose during your program.

But the next step is what really counts.

Burning fat and building muscle! After the excess glucose is utilized, then the body starts to burn fat, which burns at a much slower rate than glucose. So although the scale moves down much slower, don't be discouraged. Good work is being accomplished!

Training is key in weight loss, because when you exercise, you burn calories. And when you burn calories, the body must compensate for the extra energy being used, so the mitochondria inside your cells divide. Since the mitochondria act as our power plants, burning fuel, they divide as you exercise, burning twice as much. Nothing else will do that. Realize that by exercising, the body will compensate by burning more fat. It's that simple.

So are you ready to train? I'd like to provide you with a successful program to help you get started, no matter how badly you are out of shape. I've watched people who could barely lift 5 pounds move up to 30 pounds in just a couple weeks. You can do it! You must do it!

The Benefits of Exercise

Regular physical activity (30 minutes of walking or raking leaves or 15 minutes of jogging) that is performed on most days of the week reduces the risk of developing or dying from some of the leading causes of illness and death in the United States. Regular physical activity improves health in the following ways:

- Reduces the risk of dying prematurely from heart disease. A good physical workout improves the strength of all the muscles in your body, particularly your heart muscle.
- Reduces the risk of developing diabetes, as it lowers the blood sugar level.
- Reduces the risk of developing high blood pressure and helps reduce blood pressure in people who already have high blood pressure.
- Lowers triglyceride levels and raises HDL (good) blood cholesterol levels.
- Increases a person's sex drive.
- Reduces the risk of developing colon cancer. It also increases the motility of the colon and clears away constipation—just go for a walk in the morning and see!
- Helps control weight, develop lean muscle, reduce body fat, build and maintain healthy bones and joints.
- Delays the development of osteoporosis.

- Increases the detoxification rate as well as the cellular turnover.
- Reduces symptoms of anxiety and depression and fosters improvements in mood and feelings of well-being. Exercise has the marvelous ability to remove the adrenaline that gets pumped into our bloodstream through stress, and thus it helps keep stress under control. Stress is a huge contributor to heart problems.

Physical activity also causes the release of endorphins, which in layman's terms are the body's natural feel-good hormones. Exercise is also helpful in normalizing women's hormone levels, and there is evidence to suggest that women who exercise regularly have significantly fewer problems with PMS, menopause, and breast cancer when compared to women who do not exercise.

IT'S TIME TO GET OFF THE COUCH!

The human body was created perfectly by God for running and walking. I am not suggesting that you need to commit yourself to spending hours on end at the local gym, but I am a proponent of breaking the lethargy syndrome that seems to bind so many people I meet. You were not designed by God to come home at the end of the day and plop down in front of the television for the last hours of the day after having sat at a desk for 8+ hours. Your body was not made for inactivity while you pour in the calories with a poor diet. It's a recipe for disaster.

Check out the following chart from the *Dietary Guidelines for Americans* that compares the number of calories your body burns during one hour of various activities. These statistics are based on a healthy man of 175 pounds and a healthy woman of 140 pounds.

Activity	Calories Used Per Hour	
	Man	Woman
Sitting quietly	100	80
Standing quietly	120	95
Light activity:	300	240
Cleaning house		
Office work		
Playing baseball/golf		
Moderate activity:	460	370
Walking briskly (3.5 mph)		
Cycling (5.5 mph)		

Activity	Calories Used Per Hour	
	Man	Woman
Gardening, Dancing		
Playing basketball		
Strenuous activity:	730	580
Jogging (9 min. mile)		
Playing football		
Swimming		
Very strenuous activity	920	740
Running (7 min. mile)		
Racquetball		
Skiing		

WHERE TO START?

There are countless ways to begin exercising. Any type of exercise is better than none. You do not have to become an athlete. Take your spouse's hand and head out the door for a comfortable walk, burn some calories, and perhaps put a little spark of romance in your day. Depending on the distance to your job, consider walking. Park your car at the farthest end from the store entrance and take a little stroll before going inside. Something as simple as climbing five flights of stairs every day will significantly lower your risk of heart disease. Every step you walk or run burns calories.

There are any number of exercise choices available to you. There's fast walking, jogging, cycling, swimming, weight-lifting, calisthenics, dance, hiking, skating, tennis, basketball, aerobics, martial arts, rollerblading, and on and on. Some find that a membership at a health club keeps them motivated as well as provides all the equipment they like to use. Others prefer to set up a home gym, while others stick more with an aerobic program that requires little or no equipment.

Let's face it, though—there's no shortage of exercise choices or ways to do those exercises. The question is whether we make health and fitness a priority in our lives.

BEFORE YOU START

- If you are over 40 and in poor health, a treadmill test is highly recommended. A physician or exercise specialist can provide this test that checks blood pressure and uses an electrocardiogram to monitor heart performance. Better to be safe than sorry.

- Think about your goals. Setting and meeting short- and long-term goals is a tremendous encouragement to keep developing and maintaining an exercise program. Your goal might be to achieve a target heart rate each day or to walk a certain distance, but having something to shoot at will keep you focused.
- Whatever exercise you choose, get the right equipment to help you facilitate that exercise. For instance, if you are going to walk or run, go to a shoe store that specializes in running and talk with trained personnel who know what you'll need. Saving $20 or $30 on a cheap pair of shoes isn't worth it.
- If you are really out of shape, begin your physical activity program with short sessions (5-10 minutes) of physical activity and gradually build up to the desired level of activity (30 minutes). You don't have to run marathons for your health to reap significant benefits. You just need to be consistent.
- Keep in mind that physical activity does not need to be strenuous to achieve health

benefits. The same moderate amount of activity can be obtained in longer sessions of moderately intense activities (such as 30 minutes of brisk walking) as in shorter sessions of more strenuous activities (such as 15-20 minutes of jogging).

■ Consider weather conditions. Excessive heat or cold must be seriously considered. Never put yourself at risk.

■ Drink water—before, during, and after exercise, especially during warm weather. Replacing water lost by sweating is crucial.

■ Don't overdo it. Pushing too hard can lead to damage.

■ Check with a doctor immediately if you ever have symptoms such as chest pain or pressure, heart irregularity, or unusual shortness of breath.

STRETCHING

Before starting to exercise, spend five to ten minutes doing warm-up stretching exercises, no matter how intense your workout is going to be. Properly stretching your muscles lessens the likelihood of any muscles being damaged. It is also good to spend the last five minutes of your exercise program doing the same stretching exercises to increase your flexibility.

Here are three stretches that I recommend. Do each of the warm-up activities three times.

- Hamstring stretch. The hamstrings are the big muscles in the back of your thigh. Place one foot on a chair, and the other about 18 inches away. Keep your back straight and lean your arms on the bent knee and gradually lean forward until you feel the upper part of the straight leg being stretched. Hold it for a count of 20, and then repeat with the other leg.

- Quadriceps stretch. The quadriceps muscle is on the front of your thighs. Place your left hand against a wall for balance. While standing straight, bend your right knee, bringing your foot up and back, while reaching back with your left hand to grasp the right foot. Avoid straightening the left knee completely. Grab your right ankle with your right hand and pull toward your buttocks for a count of 20. Then repeat with the other leg.

- Upper body stretch. Standing in an upright position and clasping your hands behind your back, make sure your elbows remain straight. Pull your shoulders back, and then bend forward, lifting your arms above your head, elbows still straight and hands clasped. Stand straight again and, holding your clasped hands away from your buttocks and keeping your elbows straight, twist your upper body to the right and to the left twice.

Walking Is a Wise Choice

I recommend that you consider walking as a great starting point for exercise. It brings all the health benefits listed previously, and it is a very doable exercise. Recent studies have shown that a brisk walk provides strenuous enough exercise for cardiovascular training in most adults. And unlike running, it puts little strain on your knees and legs.

Pace Yourself

As you set goals for how long you are going to exercise, keep in mind that it's okay to be a bit out of breath, but not so much that you can't talk. Pace your workout so that you push without overdoing it. If you are still tired an hour after the exercise, you should back off a bit and build up slower.

If you prefer to be more scientific about it, measure your heart rate by taking your pulse. Aim for a heart rate between 70 and 80 percent of the maximum for your age group. If you need to lose weight, you can achieve the greatest loss if you aim for about 60 percent of your maximum heart rate and exercise for 45-60 minutes three to five times a week.

Age	70-80% of Max Rate	60% of Max Rate
20	140-160	120
30	133-152	114
40	126-144	108
50	119-136	102
60	112-128	96
70	105-120	90

PRACTICAL EXERCISE TIPS

1. Schedule exercise into your family life. Write it in as if it's an important meeting.
2. Start where you are. No matter what physical shape you are currently in, you can begin some sort of exercise program. If you can't get out of the house to walk,

start by walking in place. Then, increase slowly! Every little bit helps.

3. Use what you have! You don't have to buy an expensive club membership to start exercising. You can walk or ride your bike for free! If you desire exercise instruction, check out a book or an instructional video at your local library.

4. Exercise consistently. Exercise at least three times a week for 20-30 minutes. You will be amazed at how this will help to cut your cravings and give you more energy immediately.

5. Get an exercise buddy. If you have trouble staying motivated, then get a partner to help you keep your commitment. If you have an exercise buddy, you'll be more likely to show up for exercise times. Plus, it's a lot of fun to share workouts with a friend.

6. Take advantage of everyday activities. Take the stairs instead of the elevator at work. Do this every time you go somewhere, and you'll soon discover how much these little changes make for big results.

THE ONE PERFECT DIET

AFTER COMPLETING THE *CANDIDA* CLEANSE, going on a minimum of a three-day fast (10 days would be better), and beginning an exercise program, you need to know what you can take in on a daily basis. It's not the time to go on a bender when you lose 10 pounds. It's the time to dig in and complete your course. So here are some guidelines to help you finish the race.

Did you know that God has provided a plan for everything we need, including what to eat? It's true, and God's plan is that we be submitted to Him in every area of our lives. He wants us to be free from other controls and dominion (Romans 6:14), including being in bondage to food. We've been redeemed from all bondages by the death and resurrection of Jesus Christ our Lord. I believe that He alone should have authority over our spirit, soul, and body.

We need to bring our eating under submission to God. We are spiritual beings who live in physical bodies. We are the temples of the Lord. Our body is merely a vehicle for fulfilling His purpose on the earth. Once you get that perspective, you'll eat to live, not live to eat. So before you read the following plan for eating God's way, take a moment to pray and submit yourself to God. Ask the Lord to show you areas where you can enhance your daily living by making dietary changes. He's getting ready to show you, because He wants you to have victory in this area of your life.

GOD'S ANCIENT PLAN

God had a plan for healthy eating from the very beginning. Those who follow it walk in health, and those who don't are left to struggle with malnutrition, obesity, and disease. Need proof? Studies show that Israel is the healthiest nation on the earth, while the United States is ranked a dismal 96. That statistic alone should make you stop and take notice of what God has to say about your diet.

To fulfill the Word of God, the Jews observe the laws of Kashrut (keeping Kosher) as established in the Old Testament. So many times we think of the Old Testament as a lot of do's and don'ts, but we fail to realize that God never does anything without a purpose. Those do's and don'ts have meaning! Although we will probably never know all the intricacies of the full benefits from eating God's way, I want to explore a few.

Hosea 4:6 says, "My people are destroyed from lack of knowledge. Because you have rejected knowledge, I also reject you . . . because you have ignored the law of your God." Does that mean you're not going to heaven if you do not follow the dietary laws of the Old Testament? No, of course, not. The early church made it clear that it was not a mandatory part of the Christian faith (Acts 15). But I do believe that when we disregard the wisdom that God has already provided, we lose—in this case, our health.

Fad diets work temporarily, with an 85-percent failure rate of lasting weight loss. Starving works great until you start eating again. Exercise is fantastic, but if you don't eat right, your body will still starve for proper nutrition. This will absolutely show up in one manner or another. Everything in life is about choices, so set your will toward making right ones and reap the wonderful rewards God has in store for you.

In my book, *How to Feel Great All the Time*, I devote an entire chapter to the ONE PERFECT Diet, The Levitical Diet, but for the space restrictions of this booklet, I must limit my observations. According to Leviticus 11 and Deuteronomy 14, you may eat any animal that has cloven hooves and chews its cud—cattle, sheep, goats, buffalo, and deer. It specifically excludes the hare, pig, camel, and the rock badger. Shellfish such as lobsters, oysters, shrimp, clams, and crabs are all forbidden. Fish such as tuna, carp, salmon, and herring are all permitted. For birds there is less criteria. For the birds that are forbidden, it does not specify why. However, they all are birds of prey and/or scavengers. Birds such as chicken, geese, ducks, and turkeys are all permitted.

The important point is not to get into the bondage of having to look for everything marked "Kosher," but to realize that God has given a very clear plan for the foods we should eat. For example, the laws regarding Kosher slaughter are so sanitary that Kosher butchers and slaughterhouses have been exempted from many USDA regulations. In Kosher slaughtering the method is widely recognized as the most humane method of slaughter possible. There is no pain or fear in the animal, with no chemical releases, whether natural or synthetic. In this method, there is also rapid and complete draining of the blood. The Bible specifies that we do not eat blood because the life of the animal is contained in the blood. Today we know that disease is found in the blood, and if it is not drained properly, you can ingest it into your system.

SEPARATION OF MEAT AND DAIRY

The Old Testament says that meat and dairy should never be consumed together. God had a dual purpose for a waiting time between eating meat and dairy. First, there is evidence that the combining of meat and dairy interferes with digestion. It's important to realize that the key to losing weight naturally and living healthy is dependent on good digestion and the absorption of nutrients. Whatever inhibits digestion needs to be avoided.

Plus, it is no coincidence that it takes approximately three hours to digest fish and fowl and anywhere from six to eight hours to digest meat. Why extend that time with milk? No modern food preparation technique can reproduce the health benefit of the Kosher law of eating them separately.

Remember that anything from an animal is high in fat, so eat more fowl and fish and less red meat. They take less time to digest, which means more energy for you and less energy devoted to processing a large piece of meat. Stick with Kosher if possible. If Kosher is not available, go for the hormone-free.

THE EXCELLENCE OF FISH

According to Leviticus 11:9, fish is considered to be a clean food. It is naturally low in calories and rich in health-giving oils as well as essential vitamins and minerals. Fish contain important Omega-3 fatty acids, which have been proven to lower cholesterol, inhibit blood clots, lower blood pressure, and reduce the risk of heart attack and stroke. Researchers at Rutgers University have shown that fish oil is also an effective cancer fighter, reducing your risk of breast, pancreatic, lung, prostate, and colon cancers. The best fish sources are salmon, mackerel, and halibut.

Step-by-Step Program

The following is a step-by-step program to reduce your weight. With the emphasis on making the noon meal your main meal of the day, it may require that you rearrange your schedule a bit to prepare your food ahead of time. Don't be discouraged, though. Think of it as though you're simply packing a lunch box before you leave home!

- When you first awake, drink 6-8 ounces of *Clustered Water*™.

- Within 10-15 minutes take two ounces of *Body Oxygen*™.

- Wait at least 15-20 minutes before taking in anything else.

- In a blender, mix one cup of yogurt without added sugar, one freckled banana, 6 ounces of apple juice, soy or rice milk, one heaping scoop of *Creation's Bounty*, and fill the balance with a few ice cubes and distilled water. Drink as much as you like, then continue to drink it throughout the morning. Feel free to substitute any other fresh fruit that blends well, such as strawberries or peaches without added sugar.

- While you have the shake on your stomach, you may want to try an ephedra-free energy supplement with plenty of B vitamins included. I recommend "4-weight-loss."

- Every day drink half your body weight in ounces of water. Feel free to drink more if you'd like.

- Midmorning, have a fresh piece of fruit, preferably a type of melon in season.

- Approximately 15 minutes before you are planning to eat lunch, such as when you begin the meal preparation, eat five almonds. This will send a signal to the brain telling you that you are full.

- For lunch, have a piece of broiled or baked fish, or tuna without the mayo (you can substitute plain yogurt in tuna salad), or baked or broiled chicken. You can also have two boiled eggs as a substitute for your meat protein. Eggs are especially convenient when you are on the go. Add steamed veggies and rice, and one large salad with olive oil and apple cider vinegar for your dressing. Then add your favorite herbs. This is a guideline for your daily lunch. Make it your biggest meal. While eating, take a digestive enzyme.

- If possible, don't eat at exactly the same time every day. Eat when you are hungry! When you eat at the same time every day, the brain will send a signal to your stomach to empty, and it will seem hungry even if it is not. By eating at different times each day, you will learn to eat when you are truly hungry.

- Somewhere between 2:00 and 3:00 P.M., take one ounce of *Body Oxygen*™ along with another 6 ounces of *Clustered Water*™.

- Throughout the afternoon or at your afternoon break, eat three fresh fruits and veggies, such as carrot sticks, celery sticks, apples, grapes, cucumbers, etc.

- Sometime before 6:00 P.M. (remember, the later you eat, the more food gets retained unburned overnight) have one cup of brown rice, a sweet potato or two red potatoes along with some lentils, red or black beans, and a piece of salmon two or three nights a week. Season with all the onions, garlic, and a bit of extra virgin olive oil that you want. Have two servings of steamed vegetables, such as cabbage, broccoli, artichokes, beets, green beans, etc. You may use sea salt or Vege-Sal to season, but no more than 1/2 teaspoon. And eat the salad last! The living enzymes in the fresh vegetables eaten last work to break down all the other foods just eaten. Take a digestive enzyme with your meal.

■ One or two cups of herbal tea without sweeteners are fine throughout the day, hot or cold.

■ Right before going to bed, eat 1/2 cup of pure oat bran (proven to cut your risk of cancer by 30 percent) with soy or rice milk. Along with the oat bran, take 2 to 4 "Colon Cleanse" capsules. It is very effective in the elimination of waste from the bowels.

■ Fresh fruit and vegetable juices are allowed before 3:00 P.M. These must be fresh— not canned, frozen, or processed.

■ Each month plan a three-day fast!

As you can see, there are a lot of foods you can eat. But they are the right foods—pure and unprocessed. Your body can easily digest and assimilate these foods and use them to work on healing the body, instead of expending all your energy breaking down the wrong foods. Making the daily right choices is the key to success! I believe you will choose the right foods at the right time. Ask the Holy Spirit to help you as you retrain yourself to choose wisely.

PRACTICAL TIPS

■ Wait 10-15 minutes before having a second helping. This is how long it takes to get the signal to the brain to tell you you're full. In doing this, you usually won't want a second helping.

■ After your dinner, take a brisk walk. If your health does not allow it yet, start with walking in place for 5-10 minutes and increase as you can.

■ Don't drink anything with your meals. If you must drink, have water with a slice of lemon. Sodas, teas, and coffees interfere with the stomach acids and enzymes vital for digestion.

■ If you have a problem with poor digestion, try a glass of steam-distilled water with a teaspoon of raw honey, a fourth of a fresh lemon, and two tablespoons of organic apple-cider vinegar. This mixture can be taken with each meal and has been proven to increase your digestive ability.

- Eat as many *fresh fruits and vegetables* a day as possible. By eating five per day, according to Johns Hopkins University, you can cut your risk of cancer by 30 percent, lower your systolic blood pressure by 5.5 points and the diastolic pressure by 3.0 points, and reduce your risk of heart disease by 15 percent and the risk of a stroke by 27 percent.

- Go to your local health food store and get a good powdered kelp to use for your seasoning. This is a great additive to your food as well as a plus to the thyroid, which controls your entire metabolism. A liquid bladder wrack—an old herbal remedy used for low thyroid—is also excellent when on a weight-loss program. It's very natural to the body and excellent for weight loss by speeding up the metabolism with no harmful side effects.

- Stay away from processed foods and go for foods rich in color. Stay away from the white deadly things! White sugar, white flour, white salt, even white potatoes. Choose red potatoes instead of white. Choose a dark lettuce or spinach instead of iceberg. Try to eat foods that are as close to the way that God created them—chemical free!

■ Think about sprouting at home. It's easy, it's fun, it's cheap, and it tastes good! Even the kids love them and love to grow them! They're great on sandwiches and salads, and they can be used as snacks as well. The rewards are great. They are loaded with trace minerals that are not so easily found in other foods. You can get everything you need at your local health food store to sprout.

■ Go for Bible snacks instead of the processed foods. Fresh fruits, fresh veggies, nuts, raisins, granolas, yogurts, unrefined crackers, and flat breads—get creative! Genesis 43:11 specifically mentions pistachios and almonds. That's interesting in that those are particularly low in fat and calories. Nuts in general are a great snack food, with the exception of peanuts, which are really not a nut! Nuts are naturally rich in zinc, copper, iron, calcium, magnesium, and phosphorus, as well as being high in protein.

■ Yogurt, or fermented milk, isn't mentioned in the Bible, but according to history we know that it was a mainstay at that time. It is the ideal diet food for folks who want to add flavor and health benefits to their diet. Be sure not to get the yogurt with artificial sweeteners or with added sugars. Yogurt is a natural antibiotic that keeps your digestive system healthy by replacing the good flora in the intestinal track. This is needed for a healthy immune system. You can use yogurt in a variety of ways with salad dressings.

■ Extra virgin olive oil is by far the best oil you can use! It has been proven to be the healthiest for your heart. It helps to lower your cholesterol level instead of clogging your arteries the way the saturated fats found in your typical grocery store oils and margarineated butter do. It is far more versatile and can be used for just about anything. Medicinally speaking, olive oil has proven to be a natural antibiotic as well as antiviral. It tastes great and is good for you!

Practical Application

Putting the ONE PERFECT Diet into your daily living is actually very easy once you get in the swing of things. The important key is to get the body back into a place of homeostasis, which is a happy, healthy body, and the proper foods will make a world of difference. The rewards of healthy living, an energetic body, and sound, clear thinking will cause you to never want to turn back.

Remember that God's way works!

Step by step, it is possible to regain and maintain your perfect weight. There is no substitute for cleaning your body of toxins and restoring health throughout your entire system. And there's no substitute for exercise and a perfect diet that delivers all the nutrients your body requires. If you listen to God's voice and follow His plan, He will help you get where you really want to be—whole in every way!

VALERIE SAXION'S
SILVER CREEK LABS

THROUGHOUT THIS BOOKLET, I HAVE NOTED FOUR PRODUCTS that will aid you in your weight-loss efforts as well as promote a healthy body. To order these products or to contact Silver Creek Laboratories for a complete catalog and order form of other nutritional supplements and health products, call (817) 236-8557, or fax (817) 236-5411, or write us at:

> 7000 Lake Country Dr.
> Fort Worth, TX 76179

Body Oxygen. A pleasant-tasting nutritional supplement that is meticulously manufactured with cold pressed aloe vera. The aloe is used as a stabilized carrier for numerous nutritional constituents, including magnesium peroxide and pure anaerocidal oxygen, hawthorne berry, ginkgo biloba, ginseng, and St. John's Wort. It helps naturally fight infections, inflammation, and degeneration by taking oxygen in at the cellular level. It also commonly helps in colon cleansing, regular elimination, and provides a feeling of increased energy and mental alertness.

Candida Cleanse. A decade in coming, this is the most powerful natural agent I know of in the fight against *Candida*. It is specifically formulated for TOTAL *Candida* cleansing. A two-part system is also available to rid the body of *Candida* and parasites called *ParaCease*.

Dr. Lorenzen's Clustered Water is probably the greatest breakthrough in health science product development in this century. Clustered Water, produced at home using one ounce of solution to one gallon of steam-distilled water, replenishes the most vital support for all cellular DNA and the 4,000 plus enzymes that are involved in every metabolic process in your body. This amazing product increases nutrient absorption by up to 600 percent, which means your vitamins and organic foods will deliver far more vital nutrients to your body. It replicates the powerful healing waters of the earth! Excellent for cleaning out lymphatic fluids! It comes in a

C-400 formula for those who are generally healthy and detoxed, and a SBX formula for the immune-compromised.

Creation's Bounty. Simply the best, pleasant-tasting, green, whole, raw, organic food supplement available—a blend of whole, raw, organic herbs and grains, principally amaranth, brown rice, spirulina, and flaxseed. This combination of live foods with live enzymes assists your body in the digestion of foods void of enzymes. You will gain vital nutrients, protein, carbohydrates, and good fats to nourish your body and brain, resulting in extra energy and an immunity boost as well. It is a whole food, setting it apart from other green foods on the market.

Unleash Your Greatness

AT BRONZE BOW PUBLISHING WE ARE COMMITTED
to helping you achieve your **ultimate potential**
in functional athletic strength, fitness, natural
muscular development, and all-around superb
health and youthfulness.

Our books, videos, newsletters, Web sites, and training seminars will bring you the very latest in scientifically validated information that has been carefully extracted and compiled from leading scientific, medical, health, nutritional, and fitness journals worldwide. **Our goal is to empower you!** To arm you with the best possible knowledge in all facets of strength and personal development so that you can make the right choices that are appropriate for *you.*

Now, as always, **the difference between greatness and mediocrity** begins with a choice. It is said that knowledge is power. But that statement is a half truth. Knowledge is power only when it has been tested, proven, and applied to your life. At that point knowledge becomes wisdom, and in wisdom there truly is *power.* The power to help you choose wisely. **So join us** as we bring you the finest in health-building information and natural strength-training strategies to help you reach your ultimate potential.